My Persona

*Gareth's Big Cycling Adventure
from Land's End to John O'Groats*

Gareth Lyon

Dedication

I would like to thank quite a few people who helped me along this journey. Firstly I'd to thank Helen, my wife, and my two lovely daughters, Grace and Evelyn. They allowed me to take the time out to prepare and do these crazy challenges. I love you all to the moon and back.

Secondly I'd like to thank my dad, William Lyon, for his support throughout my life and before, during and after the ride. He jumped at the chance to help and fed and watered me well. He was brilliant company especially when the going got tough.

Thirdly I would like to thank my fellow riders from both the Land's End to John O'Groats and the Jonathan Curwen Memorial rides. Although I did do the first ride solo (mainly), I really enjoyed the time and appreciated the support of Jez Scaiff, Paul Evans and Iain Ritson. The Wales ride was a team effort with Ben Willis, Jez Scaiff and Paul Evans. You are my good friends who have supported me and hopefully enjoyed the ride.

Finally I would like to thank all of my friends and family who were very generous in supporting both the Prostate Cancer UK and The Clatterbridge Cancer Trust charities. Your generosity and words of encouragement really helped me deal with the long hours in the saddle and made the pain worthwhile.

Introduction

It all started with a crazy idea, to do an endurance challenge that would test me to the limits, to cycle from Land's End to John O'Groats. I have always had a fascination with doing this challenge but had never had the time to fit it in. In 2017 the opportunity arose and I asked my dad, at the end of April 2017 – "Do you want to be my support driver, if I were to do Land's End to John O'Groats in a couple of months". "Yes" was his immediate response! My wife Helen, asked what we were talking about and then said "He will never do it!" These were the famous last words that would inspire my journey across Britain.

I set out to do the challenge at the end of June / early July (in only 9 weeks' time) in 10 days, riding solo because I wanted to test myself both physically and mentally. My father was my support vehicle, which meant that he looked after everything to ensure that I could just focus on riding. It was also incredible to have him with me, to experience this journey together, especially when the going got tough (which it did, a lot). This book focuses on my experience of doing a supported solo ride although three friends joined me on 3 separate days to provide their moral support and their local knowledge of the area. I had to have 2 enforced rest days in the middle of the ride because we already had a ticket to see Tom Jones on the middle Saturday.

I am not a cycling expert, as I am actually more of an average running club runner than a cyclist. Before the ride I would have described myself as reasonably fit, but probably half a stone overweight. So, not a super fit athlete with the physique of a racing snake that has to run round the shower to get wet. Land's End to John O'Groats has been on my bucket list for a long time and I love a challenge.

Another major motivation for the challenge was raising money for Prostate Cancer. This is a disease that affects 1 in 8 men in the UK. It has also affected my family. My uncle George has had it and thankfully was operated on and is now fully recovered. My father is also being closely monitored for the condition. Cancer was also a theme on the ride, with my friend John Stephenson being taken into palliative care. Riding for such a worthy cause became a personal mission to help improve the lives of people with cancer.

I have divided the book into these sections: before the ride (which includes tips on training, planning and preparations), the ride (which is a journal of the journey), after the ride (practicalities and feelings), A Long and Winding Road – the lessons from my big cycling adventure, Epilogue: The Jonathan Curwen Memorial ride around Wales, maps of the ride and photos of the ride.

This book is not intended to be an encyclopaedia of knowledge on Land's End to John O'Groats but is hopefully interesting, practical and perhaps useful for ordinary people (like me) considering this challenge. It could inspire others to do something similar and/or provide practical tips on how to go about it.

I completed the Land's End to John O'Groats cycle ride (975 miles) in aid of Prostate Cancer UK and it was absolutely amazing. It was an almost spiritual experience for me and one I will never forget. I have since cycled 670 miles around Wales (in aid of the Clatterbridge Cancer Charity) in memory of my good friend Jonathan Curwen.

Before the Ride

Planning the route

There are many different answers on the internet on how far it is between Land's End to John O'Groats, ranging from 814 miles (using minor roads in places) and 837 miles (using main roads and Google maps). The problem is that both of these routes use motorways, where cyclists are not permitted.

The minimum distance, by road, where cycling is permitted is 874 miles (as is shown on the signs at Land's End and John O'Groats).

I scoured the internet for route plans and also bought a book, "Land's End to John O'Groats, Self Help Cycle Guide, written by Royston Wood, for routes and other guidance. There were multiple route options but generally the routes were pretty similar.

Several factors influenced the planning of the route:

- I wanted to do the ride over 10 days
- I wanted to enjoy the ride, so it wasn't about finding the shortest route
- I needed to book accommodation at reasonable rates
- I wanted to stay at home, in Tarporley, Cheshire, after 4 days, so had to plan the route to take in enough miles before / after arriving on day 4

- I tried to keep my mileage between 80 and 110 miles per day, so I could maintain momentum
- I wanted to minimise the climbing because I am not an expert cyclist
- I wanted to avoid the busier main roads where possible

I used Strava route builder (www.strava.com) to create my routes. This is an excellent tool that allowed me to change my routes, minimise my elevation gain and consider landmarks I wanted to take in along the way. Strava also allows you to download the routes to a cycling sat nav device (more on this later).

I planned the route 4 or 5 times before I was happy and had accommodation booked. In the end my planned route was 944 miles, with a maximum daily mileage of 118 and a minimum of 82 miles, with just over 49,000 feet elevation gain. I ended up planning to zig zag Scotland (mid to East Coast to West Coast to East Coast) to take in the scenery and minimise the climbing.

My planned route

Here is the route that I planned to take.

Day	Start / End Points	Elevation gain (ft)	Miles	Cumulative	Comments
1	Land's End to Okehampton	7,184	105	105	Easily the hardest climbing day and I tried to avoid the busy A30.
2	Okehampton to Bristol	6,324	99	204	I had intended to go to Bath but the mileage was too high.
3	Bristol to Leominster	5,413	85	289	I added in the scenic Malverns to increase the mileage.
4	Leominster to Tarporley	3,247	82	371	This was to be my shortest day, back home.
5	Tarporley to Kendal	3,421	92	463	This was mainly on main roads, limiting the climbing.
6	Kendal to Moffat	3,897	88	551	This was mainly on main roads, limiting climbing.
7	Moffat to Perth	4,744	94	645	This took in the Scottish Borders / Edinburgh.
8	Perth to Kinlochleven	4,686	95	740	This took in stunning scenery of the Highlands.
9	Kinlochleven to Tain	5,160	118	858	This was to be the longest day, but was the penultimate day, so I figured I could cope.
10	Tain to John O'Groats	5,090	86	944	A short day, mileage wise, but lots of climbing.

Although I had a planned route there was always some flexibility allowable, as most of the accommodation was booked without a cancellation fee and I was going to be accompanied by 3 friends on separate days, whose local knowledge was used to adjust the route.

Accommodation

I was travelling with my father (my support vehicle) so I tried to book twin room accommodation throughout, with an Ensuite bathroom. I was also trying to book accommodation as close to my planned route as possible, but some adjustment was required, both to the accommodation and the route. I was keen to have some flexibility so tried to avoid accommodation with cancellation charges where possible.

I ended up booking the following types of accommodation:

- Pubs with rooms (generally good facilities but noisy)
- Bed and Breakfasts (Relatively inexpensive, fabulous hospitality but some came with shared bathrooms)
- Hotels (great facilities, food and Ensuite bathrooms, but more expensive)
- A bunk house hostel (terrible facilities, shared bathrooms and we had to use our own towels)
- I needed secure storage facilities for my bike
- I needed a good breakfast included, preferably with porridge, to set me up for the day
- I needed drying facilities for my kit (I had two sets of everything so would hand wash (in the shower) the set I had worn that day and dry it overnight)

My budget was £60 - £90 per night for the room and breakfast.

Getting to the Start

I was going to a university reunion, watching the T20 cricket at Taunton, in Somerset, on the Friday before the ride, so I was almost there (only another 147 miles to go!). I caught the train from Crewe to Taunton, carrying only what I needed for the weekend. My father brought my bike and all my Land's End to John O'Groats equipment with him and picked me up from Taunton on the Sunday, the day before the ride.

We checked into our room, at a pub in Penzance, where we left the bike. Penzance was buzzing with the Golowan festival which meant lots of live music, activities for all the family and people drinking / generally enjoying themselves. It made for a great party atmosphere. How nice of them to put a party on for me!

My dad and I spent the afternoon having a nice walk along the front to Newlyn and back. It was a relaxing way to spend the last day before the big ride. I made sure I wasn't late to bed. I was excited and apprehensive, but couldn't wait to get onto the bike the following day.

On the morning of the ride my father drove me and the bike to Land's End for 8 o'clock, ready for the big cycling adventure to start.

What do I need to take with me?

I've broken this into 3 parts – what I needed on me, on the bike and in the car

On me

- Bib Shorts
- Base Layer
- Cycling Shirt
- Gilet
- Wind stop / rain stop jacket
- Socks
- Cycling shoes
- 1 litre bottle with water
- 1 litre bottle with water and 2 hydration tablets
- Helmet
- Sunglasses
- 2 SIS Energy Gels (1 per hour)
- 1 Clif Energy Bar (1 per 2 hours)
- Garmin Vivoactive Watch
- Factor 30/50 sun cream
- Bum cream (apply before cycling!)

On the bike

- 2 inner tubes
- 2 Co2 canisters
- Co2 inflator or mini hand pump
- Saddlebag – medium size to fit tools and 2 tubes
- Dry Bag for mobile (essential on wet days)
- Garmin Explorer 820 cycling sat nav
- Front light
- Back light
- Small factor 50 sun cream
- 2 Tyre levers
- Multitool
- Money (just in case)
- Mobile battery power pack / charger cable

In the car

- Bib Shorts
- Base Layer
- Cycling Shirt
- Gilet
- Wind stop / rain stop jacket
- Socks
- Bum cream
- Energy Bars
- Energy Gels
- SIS Energy / recovery drink
- Oil
- Rags for cleaning and lubricating the bike
- 40 litre water bowser
- Normal food and drink
- Camping stove for hot drinks and soup
- Stand pump
- Hydration tablets
- Chargers
- Factor 50 Sun cream

Training

There were many questions that I asked myself when training for the Land End to John O'Groats challenge, such as:

- How the hell do you train to cycle nearly 100 miles every day for 10 days?

- Should you taper down your training as you approach the ride?

- How can I incorporate the training into my daily routine?

- Can I cycle 100 miles in a day (I had previously only ridden 85 miles in one day)?

- How can I ensure I have the right nutrition to help my training?

Let's cover each of these questions.

How the hell do you train to cycle nearly 100 miles every day for 10 days?

I am not sure that you can fully prepare your body to cycle 100 miles per day consistently for a decent stretch of time. I had never cycled 100 miles in one day, never mind doing this day after day. How would my legs and mind cope? However, I did a few things to help:

- I built the mileage up steadily over time (although not perfectly, due to real life being a factor). This is something that I learned from running. Don't try to up your mileage too quickly because you generally get injured. However, I didn't have a long time to train for the ride!

- I did some longer rides to ensure I could go the distance, including a 100 mile ride a week before the ride. This was absolutely essential as it allowed me to establish a comfortable pace to ride at. I would definitely recommend getting the miles in your legs before a big endurance event like LEJOG.

- I trained on tired legs to become accustomed to the feeling of being tired and to build up the muscle memory. This goes against everything that I had done as a runner previously. I was accustomed to training hard and then resting, allowing the body to recover. But I didn't have the time to rest and certainly wouldn't have this luxury on the ride. This did show me that although my legs were tired, that after 15-20 miles of riding they loosened up nicely. Again, this gave me some confidence to fight through the initial pains of the day's riding.

- Do lots of climbing hills on the bike to build the legs up. As I was not an expert cyclist I was sometimes intimidated by large hills. I needed to get some big hills under my belt and learn how to climb on the bike (as there would be plenty on LEJOG).

- I spent a lot of time in the saddle, for the following reasons:

    - To ensure my backside could cope with lots of hours on the bike

    - I discovered that staying seated whilst climbing is an essential way of preserving energy. I also found that seated climbing tended to be quicker than getting out of the saddle (as I am not an elite athlete).

I was also given advice that I would get fitter on the ride. This absolutely turned out to be correct, thankfully.

Should you taper down your training as you approach the ride?

Being a runner I am accustomed to tapering my training as I approach a race, but doing Land's End to John O'Groats isn't a race – it is a test of endurance – becoming accustomed to riding with a tired body (and mind). I was therefore in two minds about tapering down but my options were limited because my preparation and training time (9 weeks) was limited.

I went for a compromise – I tried to increase my mileage right up to the challenge, but I also didn't ride for the 3 days before the ride so my legs felt fresh for the first day. I also used a weeks' holiday in Wales (4 weeks from the challenge) as a training week where I really upped the mileage and the hill climbing and got used to training on tired legs.

How can I incorporate the training into my daily routine?

I ended up cycling 2-4 times a week in my training schedule. But with hindsight I would have done 1-2 more rides a week if I could have. However fitting so many rides around real life is very difficult. However, if you are able to commute to work then this can help you to get enough rides in. But always try to get at least one longer ride in per week (over 50 miles at least). My advice is to try to do what you can, especially on tired legs, as you need to be accustomed to this on the ride.

Can I cycle 100 miles in a day (I had previously only ridden 85 miles in one day)?

Given that I was committing myself to cycle around 100 miles a day for 10 days – could I actually do 1 day? I had previously twice cycled the Great Yorkshire Bike Ride from Wetherby to Filey. This is 74 miles and I did it twice with very little training on a bike (and I cycled onto Scarborough on one occasion, making it up to 85).

I therefore did some training to get to 100 miles, and built up from 75 miles to 80 (in my Wales training week), right up to doing 100 miles in a day in the last week before the challenge. This helped me to identify neck pain as more of a problem than my legs but also gave me great confidence. I reckon (with hindsight) that if you can cycle 70-80 miles then you can cycle for another couple of hours to get to 100 miles.

How can I ensure I have the right nutrition to help my training?

I started by analysing the number of calories I needed to replace (roughly 600 calories per hour), as a result of increasing my exercise and mileage. I also consulted books, the internet, asked bike shop staff and friends their advice.

I realised after a while that I was actually overeating, as I was really upping the mileage but my weight was staying exactly the same when I did want to lose some weight to save me dragging it around. After trial and error, I realised I was eating too many energy bars and then got myself into a routine of taking one energy gel per hour and one energy bar every two hours. I also realised that it was as important to take in as much normal food as possible to ensure a balanced diet.

Hydration wise I used SIS Isotonic tablets and would have a 1 litre bottle of water and a 1 litre bottle of isotonic water (2 tablets) and got accustomed to drinking 2 litres of this combination over 3-4 hours (depending on the weather conditions).

Training – My Training Schedule

Although I wanted to gradually build up the mileage, real life does get in the way, so you have to fit in what training you can. Here is the training that I managed to complete before the ride.

Training schedule	Week 9	Week 8	Week 7	Week 6	Week 5	Week 4	Week 3	Week 2	Week 1
Ride 1	32	20	15	31	18	42	23	100	10
Ride 2		40	15	44	18	20	32	17	60
Ride 3				19	75	79	17	20	32
Ride 4									25
Total	32	60	30	94	111	141	72	137	127
2 week average		*46*	*45*	*62*	*103*	*126*	*107*	*105*	*132*
% increase			*-2%*	*38%*	*65%*	*23%*	*-15%*	*-2%*	*26%*
Cumulative miles	32	92	122	216	327	468	540	677	804

Weeks -5 and -4 were my training week in Wales, where I really upped the miles and the climbing.

Getting the bike (and navigation) ready

Servicing the bike

My 2007 Trek SLR (yes it was a 10-year old bike when I did the challenge) has been a good servant to me over the years. I did however need to make sure that it was up to the task of cycling nearly 1,000 miles in 10 days. I had my bike serviced twice before the challenge. I had it serviced as I started my training and then had a final (just to make sure) service 1 week out from the challenge. During those two services I had 2 new tyres, 1 new wheel, 2 brake blocks, 1 new derailleur, 1 new chain and new handlebar tape. Getting the bike up to scratch gave me peace of mind for the task ahead.

Neck pain problem / a late bike fit

I experienced a lot of neck pain as I upped my mileage. After speaking to a number of people I discovered that neck pain is not uncommon, especially for cyclists that increase their mileage quite dramatically (as I had done).

However, I tried to rectify this, when one week before the challenge I decided to get a bike fit to check that my bike was set up correctly for me. In the bike fit it was shown that I was hunched up, was overstretching my legs and wiggling too much in the saddle. I therefore needed to move my seat down by about an inch to straighten up my riding position (to reduce the strain on my neck) and to reduce the overstretching / wiggling. Unfortunately, my seat post (carbon) was not going to shift, so we ended up turning the handlebar post upside down and increasing that height by an inch.

Although this wasn't ideal it did have the desired effect of straightening me up and reducing my neck pain. With hindsight I really should have had the bike fit done much earlier in my training / preparations.

Navigation

I was nervous about getting lost along the way, so I had to work out how I was going to navigate the route. I didn't want to invest in a cycling sat nav because of the cost. I therefore tried a number of apps on my mobile as part of my training such as:

- Strava

- Komoot

- IPhone Maps app (standard map apps with iPhones)

The apps were useful but I found that they drained the battery life of the phone – in a 1 hour and 15-minute stint I found my battery life reducing by 40%. So without a battery pack constantly charging the phone (not advisable in wet weather), I decided I needed to invest in a dedicated cycling sat nav device.

After considerable research I decided to buy a Garmin 820 Explorer. This provides turn by turn navigation, as well as being able to record the ride (although I also have a Garmin Vivoactive Watch that records the ride and my heart rate and calories). I chose the Explorer because I didn't want the Performance pack that provides more detailed analytics such as cadence. I already have a lot of performance features on my watch (except for cadence) so it didn't warrant the additional investment.

The Garmin 820 explorer is a great piece of kit that can take downloads of the Strava maps and provide turn by turn navigation.

Social Media and raising money for charity

Because this was a really big thing for me I wanted to record it for myself and for other people to follow my progress. I also wanted to use this as an opportunity to raise money for a worthwhile cause.

A major motivation for the challenge was raising money for Prostate Cancer. This is a disease that affects 1 in 8 men in the UK. It has also affected my family. My uncle George has had it and thankfully was operated on and is now fully recovered. My father is also being closely monitored for the condition. Cancer was also a theme on the ride, with my friend John Stephenson being taken into palliative care. Riding for such a worthy cause became a personal mission to help improve the lives of people with cancer.

My wife and I decided to set up a Facebook group called Gareth's big cycling adventure. This was intended to be my diary / live feed of events and photographs from the trip. I got an awful lot of encouragement from the Facebook group and it helped me to get through some really difficult times. The ride section of this book contains extracts from my diary and photo updates.

My wife and I set up a Justgiving page so people could donate money directly to Prostate Cancer, whilst also getting the benefit of Gift Aid for the charity. I would also add offline donations to the page (without Gift Aid) when people gave me money towards the cause. My wife and I also ensured that the Justgiving page was always visible on my Facebook group

The Ride

During the ride there was a regular checklist / set of practical rules that were very useful:

- Get out early enough so that you are not cycling late into the evening
- Clean your chain and lube the bike daily – this will ensure slick gear changes
- Check tyre pressure before each ride – I pumped up to 120 psi (the max for my tyres) per day, but there are different schools of thought on this. 100-120 psi works.
- Take 2 energy gels and 1 energy bar for each 2-hour stint, although they can get a little sickly after a while
- Have 2 litres of water at all times (1 with 2 hydration tablets in), just in case you get lost or miss your stops with your support vehicle
- Wear sunscreen, Butt Cream, gloves and a helmet
- Get used to having damp clothes – if it rains you will either be wet, drying out or about to get wet, or your clothes may not be fully dry from being hand washed on the previous night
- Have set stopping points to help break up your day and know where you are meeting your support driver
- Check your route for the day and know where your hills are
- Don't burn yourself out / pace yourself
- Eat normal food at each stop but don't overeat

- Keep your stops to 15-20 minutes so that your legs don't get stiff
- Hydrate yourself, especially when it is raining or when you are feeling tired
- Stretch off at the end of each day
- Give your legs a rub down at the end of the day, or get someone else to do this for you.

Day 1 – Land's End to Okehampton

Weather: 16°C, Cloudy, 4mph E Wind
Miles: 107
Time: 7 hours and 1 minute
Elevation Gain: 7,400 ft
Moving Speed: 15.6 mph
Cumulative Miles: 107

The big ride was eventually here! I was nervous but excited about the day ahead. But my first thought was that I need to shave my legs, ready for the big challenge.

I know that cyclists do shave their legs but I have never done this before. But would it really make a difference? So, I set about shaving my legs, not very well, at first. My dad was laughing at me for 1.) Shaving my legs and 2.) For leaving it until an hour before we were due to set off.

However, after having beautifully shaved legs (bottom half only, where the cycling shorts didn't cover), we went for a hearty full breakfast to set us up for the day.

We drove to Land's End and were there just after 8am. After my dad got over the shock of having to pay £3 for all day parking (when we were only going to be there for 45 minutes), we got the bike off the car and proceeded to the sign post for the obligatory photographs to mark the start of the big cycling adventure.

The first day, from Land's End to Okehampton, was always going to be the most difficult climbing wise. Cornwall is very lumpy. However, I was setting off with fresh legs and a heck of a lot of determination.

The first leg of the journey involved cycling back down the road we had just driven down, back to Penzance and then onto St Michael's Mount, where I had my picture taken by an America tourist. After that it was over to Redruth for my first stop with my dad. However, my dad was actually behind me, so we organised a stopping point after Redruth. The first leg was 2 hours and 40 minutes and I'd covered 40 miles, so I was making good progress.

After my first stop it was on to Wadebridge and Launceston, taking in Bodmin Moor along the way. The climb from Wadebridge to the top of Bodmin Moor was relentless. 13 miles long and 1,000 feet of climbing. I did stop in Launceston to take pictures of the castle and the pretty market square.

My second stop was at the top of Bodmin Moor. My dad was getting used to making sandwiches and soup and seemed to be getting into the swing of it, if not getting a bit stressed out about exactly where we were meeting. We'd decided on a two stop strategy for the day, so our finishing pint for the day was the pretty town of Okehampton.

On the way to Okehampton was a lot more climbing and getting lost a little bit (even though I had the Garmin sat nav and route set out). For some reason I couldn't get into

Okehampton itself and ended up circling around a bit before asking a chap for directions.

On my arrival in Okehampton I was greeted by my dad with a "where the bloody hell have you been? I've been worried about you". Bless him. Our good friends Martin and Sue were also there to welcome me at the end of my first day. They happened to be house / pet sitting around 20 miles away. They gave me a very useful gift – an industrial sized bum cream applicator (a mastic gun). This could be very handy for the rest of the ride.

We stayed in a lovely and quiet B&B. The hosts were very friendly and we had a spacious twin room, with my bike stored securely in the shed.

After a protein shake (to help my muscles recover), a shower and washing my cycling gear (in the shower) we walked down to the local pub for beer (carbohydrates) and a pub dinner. This is the life! Martin and Sue were great company as always. We didn't have a late night as I was tired and needed my beauty sleep.

Day 2 – Okehampton to Bristol

Weather: 16°C, Cloudy, 6 mph SE wind
Miles: 105 miles
Time: 6 hours and 55 minutes
Elevation Gain: 4,500 ft
Moving Speed: 15.3 mph
Cumulative Miles: 212

Day 2 was planned to be a day with 99 miles ahead, and 4,400 feet of climbing, a lot less than day 1.

I had porridge for breakfast, a special request and much better to release energy for longer over the morning than a full English (although my dad was enjoying the hospitality!).

My legs felt tired but I felt sure they would soon be warmed up by the climb out of Okehampton. I was cycling through the rolling countryside of Devon and the first part of the day involved a fair bit of climbing and getting lost around Tiverton, where I had organised to meet my dad, for our first rendezvous. At the first lunch stop I had covered 37 miles in 2 hours 25 minutes, at a reasonable pace of 15 miles per hour. The climb out of Okehampton was a tough way to start and I'd climbed 2,000 feet in the first leg. I ended up getting lost in Tiverton. This meant that I would clock over 100 miles for the day.

The second leg of the day was hard work. It wasn't particularly hilly, but it was tough. I covered 38 miles in 2 and a half hours and needed a good stretch / lie down at the end of this leg. I also had a full fat coke that seemed to revitalise me.

The last leg was only 27 miles, but was going to take in the Mendip Hills, passing close to Cheddar Gorge. The Mendip Hills were absolutely beautiful, if not more climbing. Once I passed over the other side I was desperate to get to Bristol, but my route seemed to take me quite out of the way, off the road a little (but still ok for a road bike thankfully).

I did eventually arrive in the bustling city of Bristol. I have worked here a bit over the years and like the energy and vibrancy of the city. We stayed in a B&B, which was clean enough, but not a patch on the last place. I had a good soak in the bath – to ease the muscles a little, as I was pretty stiff.

We decided to find a pub (The Cottage Inn) on the waterside, at Bristol marina. On the way there and back we passed some fabulous street art on buildings and billboards. Pie, chips and a couple of pints (more carbohydrates!) for tea. Not a late one.

Day 3 – Bristol to Leominster

Weather: 14°C, Heavy Rain, 8 mph E wind
Miles: 85
Time: 6 hours and 11 minutes
Elevation Gain: 3,386 ft
Moving Speed: 14.2 mph
Cumulative Miles: 297

Day 3 was a relatively short / "easy" day, with 84 miles scheduled to Leominster, Herefordshire. However, my legs were very stiff and it was chucking it down. I fancied a cycle round the sights of Bristol before heading north. First stop was Ashton Gate stadium, the home of Bristol City Football Club, which was down the road from our B&B.

After that I did a few circuits of Bristol. Unfortunately, this was not deliberate. I discovered that the Garmin sat nav wasn't very good in built up areas and kept sending me in circles. After a short while I headed for the A38 to Gloucester just to get back on the route. Thankfully, after a few miles the sat nav synchronised and we were back in business. The first leg was awful – it just wouldn't stop raining, so much I could only see about 20 feet in front of me.

I found myself singing very loudly, as I was soaked through and struggling a bit. My go to songs were Paradise City by Guns N Roses, Gay Bar by Electric Six and The Long and Winding Road by the Beatles. An eclectic mix that was belted out at the top of my voice. God knows what the oncoming traffic made of it.

I arrived at my first stop just north of Gloucester. I'd covered 43 miles in 3 hours 22 minutes. It was pretty slow (13 miles per hour) but I did get quite lost in Bristol and it was very wet. I was quite literally washed out at the first stop and it was then that I realised that I had not drank anywhere near enough. I suppose that I had been distracted by being so wet / the persistent rain. I rehydrated and got some fuel into me for the second leg, to Leominster via Great Malvern / the Malvern hills. The rain was subsiding, thank goodness.

The Malvern Hills were a way to up the mileage (as it ended up being a dog leg of a journey) for the day and to take in some beautiful scenery. The hills around Great Malvern were pretty steep. I also had more route issues as the Garmin was trying to take me up a dirt track to the very highest point in Great Malvern. I would have struggled to climb it with a mountain bike so I declined that and decided to head towards Leominster.

On the way I had to stop at a lovely little café / art gallery. It was so posh that they didn't serve full fat Coke (or any other variety), so I ended up getting a very sugary pressed Elderflower drink, to get my energy levels back up.

I arrived in Leominster a bit broken. I was generally sore all over. I asked my dad if he could get some ice from the bar so I could have an ice bath. I then went into the ice bath and flooded the bar downstairs. My dad had also got me some cream for me to massage into my muscles. It was much needed tonight.

We had our friends Martin and Sue met us again for tea tonight. They were on their way back from Devon so we had a curry and a few beers with them. Again, it was not a late night – I was certainly not struggling to sleep on this trip.

Day 4 – Leominster to Tarporley

Weather: 12°C, Heavy Rain, 4 mph NW wind
Miles: 80 miles
Time: 5 hours and 24 minutes
Elevation Gain: 3,087 ft
Moving Speed: 15.1 mph
Cumulative Miles: 377

Day 4 meant going home to Tarporley to see the family. It also meant that my friend Jez Scaiff was going to join me and guide me through his native county of Shropshire. Jez was my much needed riding partner for the day as I had struggled a little the day before, even though it was not a very long day.

The weather was poor again as it was very wet. However, Jez really lifted my spirits and we took in lovely countryside of South Shropshire and Ludlow before heading into Shrewsbury to meet my dad for lunch. We stopped by the river near the Boathouse pub where my dad served up soup and sandwiches. Jez still goes on about his excellent Broccoli and Stilton soup to this day.

We were absolutely soaked and I changed into some slightly less damp gear for the home leg, back to Tarporley.

I could not wait to get home to see the family and to have an enforced rest for a couple of days. The rest was enforced because I had organised the ride without checking the social diary (schoolboy error). We had tickets to see Tom Jones in

Delamere forest for the middle Saturday. Compromise, rather than marriage counselling prevailed, and I was to have two days of rest and the pleasure of listening to Tom belting out some classics.

The afternoon's ride was an absolute blast. The fact that I was going home spurred me on even more.

We were met in Tarporley High Street by a welcoming committee of the mums, dads, grandparents, school teachers and some of the school children. We even had a blast of Queens "We will rock you" from my youngest daughter Evelyn on her baritone. The Chocolate shop provided some flags and balloons and we even had people donating to us from passing cars. What a reception!

Rest Day 1

My legs were in absolute pieces. I think I had either gone too hard in the second half of the day before, or it could just be that my legs were a bit tired after cycling for over 35 hours, 377 miles and climbing 18,300 feet in the last 4 days. We had also raised over £1,300 for Prostate Cancer so far.

It was a very relaxing day and my cycling gear got a proper wash in the washing machine.

Rest Day 2

My legs were still in pieces so my wife Helen decided to give me a deep tissue massage. Good god. It hurt. A lot. I had tears of pain running down my cheeks whilst my dad had tears of laughter, due to laughing at me rolling around the lounge floor.

It really hurt but it was the best thing for me and my legs felt much better afterwards.

We went to see Tom Jones that night, a few miles away in Delamere. Tom is an absolute legend and still a great performer at 77 years young. It rained (again) so we all got soaked. We had a late night, which of course is perfect preparation for a 100-mile bike ride the following day.

Day 5 – Tarporley to Bowness

Weather: 16°C, Cloudy, 12 mph NW wind
Miles: 100
Time: 6 hours and 25 minutes
Elevation Gain: 3,852 ft
Moving Speed: 15.8 mph
Cumulative Miles: 477

After 2 rest days it was time to get back on the bike, to cycle up to the Lake District. My legs felt much better for the rest and massage. The weather was nice and sunny (for possibly the first time in the trip) and the family all waved me off from home.

The first leg took me through Warrington and Wigan. I was motoring on the bike and felt strong. I passed the Warrington Wolves Rugby league ground on the way and of course stopped to take a photo. My first stop was just North of Wigan, after 33 miles.

The second leg took me to Lancaster. We stopped in the car park of a nice pub there. It was a relief to find a spot that wasn't a layby (that smelt of wee). My dad was starting to get the hang of this now. I had covered 68 miles in 4 hours and 10 minutes, at 16.3 miles per hour, so I was making good progress. I had just over 30 miles to get me to Bowness in the Lake District.

Getting close to the Lake District was fantastic as the scenery is stunning. I stopped on several occasions, once to take a picture of a heron and a few to take in the splendour of the mountains. I had also forgotten just how hilly the lakes were. I got lost a few times (again) and ended up taking some steep, unplanned diversions to get to my friend Paul's step mum's house. My dad was already there and getting everything organised.

The day had gone well. Although there were some uninspiring and busy roads and a head wind along the way I had really put my foot down and it was worth it when I reached the Lakes.

That evening we went for a walk around lovely Bowness, on Lake Windermere, and took some photos and had a Chinese meal. My friend Paul Evans joined us for dinner and was in great form, as usual. We spoke about the next day's riding, as he was going to accompany me until the half way point, leaving me in Carlisle. He had plans to take in a more scenic route, avoiding some of the busy roads with much more climbing. We leave England tomorrow on our way to Moffat. I couldn't wait to get going again.

Day 6 – Bowness to Moffat

Weather: 16°C, Cloudy, 16 mph W wind
Miles: 89
Time: 6 hours
Elevation Gain: 4,852 ft
Moving Speed: 15.1 mph
Cumulative Miles: 566

We had a relatively short day ahead, just 89 miles but Paul (king of the mountains) had plenty of climbing planned for the first half of the day. The climbing started almost as soon as we left Bowness and our first climb was Kirkstone Pass. In places this pass has a gradient of 17% (it is 1 in 4 from the other direction), rising to 1,489 feet at the top. I'll admit I may have stopped a few more times than I would normally to take photos, as it was hard work.

We made it to the top and enjoyed the views and got our breath back. The ride down the other side was just mental. It was a 25% gradient and I was struggling to keep up with Paul, who was well accustomed to riding on these roads.

Our first stop was in Greystoke, where we had lunch and checked out the Boot and Shoe Inn, which has a lot of Tarzan memorabilia. We had covered over 2,000 feet in under 2 hours. Brutal. Paul enjoyed my dad's hospitality and pointed out (about me) that "He's doing really well riding this distance on that bike!"

We set off again and thankfully we were going downhill as we left the Lakes behind. It was lovely riding in beautiful countryside. We passed two brilliant village names: Durdar (shouted out by Paul like dahdah!!) and Unthank. Both helped me to get through a tough afternoon.

As we approached Carlisle we got lost (Sat nav issues in a built up area again) and ended up following signs to the centre of Carlisle. Paul left me here and was going to nip into his office there and then cycle back to Bowness. It was fantastic to have the company of such a good rider, even if I did feel a little inadequate / inferior when I compared my standard road bike to his custom built machine.

I stopped to take some photos in Carlisle and then made my way to Scotland and to our second stop in Gretna Green. I took some photos in Gretna and met my dad for my second stop. I was quite tired as I reckon that I had gone too hard too early in the mountains. I took a caffeine energy gel as I set off to give me a boost. However, I had to stop about 5 miles on as my resting heart rate was 20 beats per minute up on what it is normally. I decided to take 15 minutes out and sit / lay on some grass to relax, stretch out and get my heart rate down. That was the last caffeine gel that I took on the whole trip.

The last leg was a tough one, but I just had to keep grinding it out. I arrived in the lovely tourist village of Moffat that is famous for having a sculpture of a ram without any ears. Although I'd climbed a fair bit during the morning my average speed for the day was a respectable 15mph. We ended up climbing 1,000 feet more than I had planned so it wasn't a surprise that I was pretty pooped that evening. We just had had pie and chips and a pint in a pub before retiring to bed in a hotel in the town square.

We hit the milestone of raising £1,500 for Prostate Cancer UK!

Day 7 – Moffat to Perth

Weather: 10°C, Very Wet, 7 mph E wind
Miles: 107
Time: 7 hours and 49 minutes
Elevation Gain: 4,790 ft
Moving Speed: 14.0 mph
Cumulative Miles: 673

I had planned a route to Perth of 84 miles but I was advised by my friend, Iain Ritson (Mr Cycling), to take a more scenic but longer route, of 107 miles. Iain knows the area as his parents live there. He frequently rides to Moffat from his home in Edinburgh. So it was only right that I took the advice of a local expert.

Oh my good lord, it hurt my face as it was raining so hard that morning. Horizontal rain would be the best description of the precipitation. There was also some decent climbing, which was good because it kept me warm. Who would have believed that this was the beginning of July! I also had a near miss coming down one of the hills. I went to grab a drink of water and when putting it back into the cradle I dropped it on the road. Thankfully I managed to miss the bottle and didn't fall off the bike. It was my first near miss of the ride.

I was meeting Iain about mid-way through the morning, in Innerleithen, where we stopped for a hot chocolate and cake. We were both absolutely frozen and soaked through. It was great to see Iain as we worked together previously and had not seen each other for a few years.

We were heading for Edinburgh first and then over the Firth of Forth and onto Perth. The weather in the afternoon did not improve at all and we had hard rain hitting us in the face all the way. Iain is a good cyclist and he shared some great tips like staying seated whilst climbing to avoid burning out. He said that standing up was the equivalent of burning matches. Thankfully I was already doing this, but it was good to reinforce my riding technique.

We stopped on the outskirts of Edinburgh, in Bonnyrigg, outside a pub where we could go to the toilet and get warm. The hot soup was very much needed as it was less than 10°C. We also received a donation from a local who was passing by and saw the Prostate Cancer sign in my dad's car. The chap said that it was a cause close to his heart. Who said the Scottish were tight!? That also lifted our spirits.

We went through Edinburgh and took in some of the sights in along the way before Iain left me to go back home. It was great having another riding partner, especially with such dreadful weather. Iain was relieved to be calling it a day and wished me luck for the rest of my journey.

It was only after I left Iain that I could take any photos because it had been so wet. I took photos of the Forth Bridges. There is one rail bridge, one road bridge and a new road bridge that was under construction. All are marvellous feats of engineering. I also received news about our friend John Stephenson, who had been taken into palliative care in Sheffield. He was suffering with cancer but his health had got much worse. It did upset but also spurred me on to take on the Forth Road Bridge.

The Forth Road Bridge is a stunning bridge. However, it is very high, exposed and it was moving a lot due to the constant traffic and the wind. Thankfully I cycled across a cycle path but it was quite unsettling and I was relieved to get to the other side. I met my dad in Inverkeithing, in possibly the worst stopping place of the whole trip, half way up a hill. I had a scotch pie and a full fat coke, but I was struggling and was cold and very tired.

After I tried to get warm again in my dad's car I got back on the bike. I wasn't in good shape and 200 yards up the road I got off the bike and had to be sick. Riding in the cold and the rain was really hard work. The last leg of that day was easily the hardest. I was exhausted and emotional. It was at this point that I decided that this was my personal Everest because it was so physically and mentally challenging. I found myself shouting "Come on", Andy Murray style and singing random tunes very loudly again. I was probably verging on delirium at points on the last leg.

Our B&B in Perth was stunning, it was almost palatial and very comfortable. It was much needed as my face was sore and red from being pelted with rain. I was so tired that I ended up eating in the B&B and getting to bed early.

This was easily the hardest day so far. The weather was brutal and I was broken for the last leg of the day. But I was determined to do it, to be able to raise money to help good friends like John, and to just keep going.

Day 8 – Perth to Kinlochleven

Weather: 14°C, Sunny, 7 mph E wind
Miles: 95
Time: 6 hours and 15 minutes
Elevation Gain: 3,832 ft
Moving Speed: 15.7 mph
Cumulative Miles: 768

I slept very well in our palatial surroundings although I was slightly nervous about today, given how tired I was after yesterday's riding. I was heading for the highlands, across to Kinlochleven, going from the East coast to the West Coast. I had deliberately chosen a longer route because I knew that the scenery today was going to be breath-taking.

I started the day with more Garmin sat nav issues. I ended up using my phone for navigation to get me onto my route. Garmin seems to struggle in built up areas, unfortunately. Thankfully it was a sunny day. I think that and the scenery helped to lift my spirits today.

Our first stop was Loch Earn, 30 miles in. It was such a lovely spot, looking over the water towards the mountains. It was a nice day, even my dad had shorts on, although they did look a little tight, possibly because of all the cooked breakfasts he'd been eating.

I left Loch Earn and then passed my first distillery of the trip. It is Scotland's oldest, the Famous Grouse distillery, just outside of Crieff. I didn't stop for a tipple though and headed through Crieff and up into the mountains. The scenery was out of this world. I was smiling every mile of the way and took loads of photos.

My second stop was at the Bridge of Orchy. We stopped at the Bridge of Orchy hotel and had a nutritious lunch of a ham and cheese roll with a full fat coke. The setting was just lovely. I had covered the last 34 miles in 2 hours and 9 minutes, so was motoring along at nearly 16 mph, even though I was loving the sightseeing.

The last leg of the day just got better. Every corner was a new photo opportunity. I did however have more navigation problems as I struggled to find our hostel in Kinlochleven. This was our first hostel of the trip. Unfortunately, this area is so popular that it is difficult to find reasonably priced accommodation. We eventually found our accommodation, up the side of a very steep hill, that I cycled up (obviously).

The accommodation was a 6 bed bunk room (with fabulous views) that I had booked out for me and my dad. It was very basic and quite a shock compared to the brilliant B&B we had left behind in Perth.

We went out for dinner at the Onich Hotel, overlooking Loch Linnhe. It was a lovely setting topped off by a pensioner on the table next to us giving us £5 towards Prostate Cancer. It was a brilliant end to such an uplifting day.

Day 9 – Kinlochleven to Tain

Weather: 21°C, Wet and Sunny, 15 mph W wind
Miles: 119
Time: 7 hours and 48 minutes
Elevation Gain: 3,898 ft
Moving Speed: 15.4 mph
Cumulative Miles: 887

We were heading back to the East coast of Scotland today. This was the longest day by far with 119 miles planned. However, I had justified doing this distance because it was the penultimate day of the big adventure. Given the length of today's ride we went for a 3 stop strategy, stopping around every 30 miles.

Unfortunately, our basic bunk room had more than me and my dad in it overnight. My dad wriggled about all night and eventually got us both up just after 5am. He had been bitten all over his legs by bed bugs. I was so tired and grumpy that I didn't give my dad much sympathy. I ended up getting on the bike just after 6am, without breakfast, but it was probably better to get out early as it was going to be a long day of riding.

The weather was shocking again, with lots of rain and not great visibility. I rode alongside Loch Leven and Loch Linnhe but the visibility meant there was no chance of me seeing Ben Nevis. Our first stop was in Spean Bridge, where I had porridge for breakfast courtesy of the camp stove my dad had (it takes him back to his army days). It rained for the whole 2 hours but I still managed to get 30 miles in, so was making good progress.

It was only on the second leg when it stopped raining and I could take my phone out of the dry-bag to take photos. Our second stop was in Invermoriston. 60 miles down in just under 4 hours. I was now approaching Loch Ness and would ride alongside it for quite a long way. It was beautiful scenery all around. As I left Loch Ness behind, at Drumnadrochit I was faced with a stupendous hill. It wasn't as high as Kirkstone pass but it was steep. I did have to stop on 3 occasions as I already had 75 miles on my legs. I also needed to get my heart rate back down again.

We stopped in Beauly at around 86 miles, after 5 hours 37 minutes in the saddle, at an average of 15 mph. Although I was going up plenty of hills I had finally found a strategy to tackle them. It had only taken 9 days to work it out (more on this in the lessons learned later). I had about 30 miles left but was doing well and actually found myself going up the gears as I was climbing, which is the opposite of what I normally do. Maybe I really was getting much fitter.

My first three legs went like a dream, but my last leg of the day was hard work. I got to 114 miles of 119 and was in a world of pain. I had chronic neck pain and had hit the wall and had nothing left in the tank. I had to stop at the side of the road, get more fuel into me and stretch / lay down for 10 minutes. I was putting my body through the wringer big time. I managed to get to our hotel in Tain, after 119 miles and just under 8 hours of riding. In total I had 2 hours without rain so I was either completely soaked through or drying out all day.

We stayed in the hotel and had steak and chips and a pint (more carbohydrates) for tea.

Day 10 – Tain to John O'Groats

Weather: 14°C, Sunny, 7 mph E wind
Miles: 88
Time: 6 hours and 4 minutes
Elevation Gain: 4,806 ft
Moving Speed: 14.8 mph
Cumulative Miles: 975

The final day of the ride. I was happy but also sad that this epic adventure is coming to an end. I was definitely looking forward to not putting on damp cycling gear the following day. It was a cool start to the day and a little breezy. It was planned to be a short day with only 85 miles, but nearly 5,000 feet of climbing ahead.

As soon as I set off it started raining. But I did 30 miles on my first leg, in 2 hours, climbing 1,000 feet. The climbing started in Golspie and I passed Dunrobin castle, which could have come out of a Disney film. I also passed through a lovely small harbour village called Brora. The Far East coast of Scotland is so beautiful and so sparsely populated. At our first stop we met up with a group of fellow LEJOGers – they took a slightly different route but watched Tom Jones, in Cartmel, in the Lakes, the night before I saw him at Delamere forest.

They were on assorted bikes and were carrying all their kit (including tents) with them as they were camping. One guy asked if he could see how heavy my bike was. He said "the heaviest thing on that is your two water bottles". I tried lifting his and could barely get the front wheel off the ground as it was a heavy bike but also had all of his gear on it (including a tent). He had owned the bike from being 14 years old. Kudos to that man for dragging that up the many hills of the ride!

The second leg involved more climbing and I would regularly pass or be passed by logging trucks. You could smell their brakes and/or clutches on the very steep inclines/descents. I was doing well on the hills but also didn't mind having 5 minutes at the side of the road admiring the views and getting the heart rate back down.

I met my dad for our last pit stop, before John O'Groats, just outside Ulbster. I had completed 60 miles in 4 hours and 9 minutes so my pace was pretty consistent. My dad was playing "Memory" by Barbara Streisand on the CD player in the car and I think he was getting a bit emotional, or he had some salt in his eye. Just 24 miles left to ride to our final destination!

I got near John O'Groats and got lost again (at least this was the last time to get lost on this trip) trying to find the sign post. After more unnecessary climbing I eventually got the end destination. I felt elated and emotional. I had put my body and mind through the wringer over the last 10 days, but, I had done it.

John O'Groats reminded me of Land's End – very isolated but with the same tourist trappings. After lots of photos and donations from very generous tourists we headed for our last B&B of the trip, near Thurso, with views out to sea.

We didn't hang around in the accommodation for too long and were taken by our hosts into the lively town of Thurso. Our hosts recommended the Y Not Bar and Grill so we headed straight there for a slap up celebratory dinner and many pints. Even though I was pretty tired I was definitely up for a party. After a dinner fit for a king we visited the pubs of Thurso. All the locals were very friendly and we played pool until the early hours.

How did the ride compare to my planned route?

I set out to do 944 miles and an elevation gain of over 49,166 feet (20,136 feet higher than Mount Everest). I ended up doing 31 miles more, but climbed 4,763 less than my planned route. My average moving speed for the whole trip was 14.8mph, which was pretty consistent except for one very wet day from Moffat to Perth.

Here is the route that I ended up taking, some of this was changed as we went along, some with the advantage of local knowledge.

Day	Start / End Points	Elevation	Minutes	Miles	Cumulative
1	Land's End to Okehampton	7,400	420	107	107
2	Okehampton to Bristol	4,500	415	105	212
3	Bristol to Leominster	3,386	371	85	297
4	Leominster to Tarporley	3,087	324	80	377
5	Tarporley to Bowness	3,852	385	100	477
6	Bowness to Moffat	4,852	360	89	566
7	Moffat to Perth	4,790	468	107	673
8	Perth to Kinlochleven	3,832	375	95	768
9	Kinlochleven to Tain	3,898	468	119	887
10	Tain to John O'Groats	4,806	364	88	975
Total		44,403	3,950	975	
Per Day		4,440	395	97.5	

In total I burned 38,000 calories, whilst riding, over the 10 days. This would explain why I lost a bit of weight across and after the trip and it also justified eating a lot more than normal on the ride.

After The Ride

The elation and the impact on my body

On my final day, even though I was tired having ridden 975 miles, I was pretty chuffed with myself and felt that a celebration was in order. My dad and I father had a brilliant (and drunken) night in a very lively Thurso. It was obvious that the adrenaline was still coursing through me, as I was in great spirits.

Saturday, the morning after – in spite of a heavy night and the miles on the bike, I felt pretty good. My legs felt fine, as they had done for the last 4-5 days. We now had to drive back home to Tarporley, in Cheshire. Just 500 miles or so.

It was on the way home that I started to realise what I had achieved. Initially we went down the roads I had cycled the day before. Some of the hills were pretty big and I knew every single turn of the road and the surrounding area. It also took us nearly 8 hours of driving to just get out of Scotland. Scotland is so long! My legs were also starting to stiffen up (and also itching to be riding). After another couple of hours, we were back in Tarporley and I couldn't wait to see my wife Helen and the girls, Grace and Evelyn.

I was met in the pub with another mini welcoming committee of Helen and the girls and a group of close friends. Everyone was really chuffed for me for completing the mammoth task and again I was surviving on adrenaline from the ride. I only had a couple of drinks and wasn't in bed too late.

On the Sunday we went to see my good friend Martin's brother, John, who had taken a turn for the worse and was now in palliative care in Sheffield. We felt compelled to see John and wanted to give Martin and his family some much needed support. It was a shock to see John so poorly, but a reunion of the gang that went on a sailing trip a few years ago did help to lift John's spirits a little. I also gave John a flash of my Wookie legs (unshaven at the top and hairless at the bottom). Despite the party atmosphere we all felt pretty emotional as we left and went for a beer and a curry.

On the way back we dropped in on my mum and dad – my mum was really proud of my achievement. We got home at around 10 that evening – pretty late given the girls were at school the following day.

On the Monday and Tuesday, I started to feel the after effects of the ride. Although my legs and muscles generally felt ok, I was physically exhausted and had to sleep for a couple of hours in the afternoon on both days. I stayed off the bike. I got weighed on Monday and had lost half a stone in weight (from 12 stone 12 pounds).

By Wednesday I was starting to come around again and I got back out on the bike and started to compile the diary of the big ride. By the end of the week I lost a further 3 pounds as my metabolism was still pretty high and I was consuming much less each day.

I was absolutely motoring on the bike

Even on my first ride back I found that I was so much quicker than I was before the challenge. My legs felt stronger and I was really taking on the hills. It is fair to say that cycling nearly 1,000 miles does make you fitter! I was absolutely motoring on the bike and was averaging 1-2 miles per hour faster and smashing my previous personal records on almost all segments of my rides (using Strava).

I am sure that this is down to me being:

- A lot fitter
- Being a better cyclist, especially hill climbing
- Being a lot leaner
- Having much stronger legs, as I had the miles in them

I did 2-3 rides a week, doing much shorter distances, with a total between 60 and 90 miles. It is fair to say that I felt good and I was also keen not to let my fitness fall off too much.

Fund Raising

Although I did the ride primarily to test myself physically and mentally, I was also raising money for Prostate Cancer UK (as this has affected my family). Throughout the ride I provided updates to my Facebook group and I would also let them know how much we had raised to date, thanking them for their wonderful generosity. On the morning after the ride I had raised £1,700. This was a real achievement as I had set a target of £500.

On the Monday, after completing the ride, I had a Facebook instant message conversation with one of my friends, John Lee. My friend was inspired by my challenge and donated £975 (£1 for each mile) to Prostate Cancer UK via his company's Give as You Earn scheme. I was completely taken aback by the amazing generosity and I did have a little cry (I couldn't help it).

The sponsorship continued and I received on and offline donations from lots of friends, colleagues and family. I think some people didn't believe that I could do it! We ended up raising over £3,250. I was absolutely staggered by everyone's generosity. I was pleased that people were inspired by my journey and also enjoyed seeing my progress and trials and tribulations along the way.

What next?

How do you follow on from cycling the length of mainland Britain, doing 975 miles in the process? It's a pretty hard act to follow, but I have thought about running a marathon (given I am more of a runner than a cyclist) or doing a triathlon.

There is a part of me that has become addicted to cycling, possibly because it has got me pretty fit and my cycling has improved a lot. However, I am not completely addicted as I am not out every single day (yet). Real life has also kicked in as I returned to being part of the family and getting back into the routine of life.

I am still undecided about what to do next, but at least I have the confidence of Land's End to John O'Groats behind me and I now know that when I set my mind to challenges I can take on almost anything. I continued to cycle through to the end of 2017, but life and work definitely got in the way.

In 2018 I ended up running a half marathon and then signing up for a marathon. Unfortunately, I got injured a fortnight before the race so couldn't run the marathon.

Early in 2019 some friends and I, over beers, decided to cycle around Wales. It's around 700 miles in 7 days, but includes 39,000 feet of climbing, which is about 1,500 feet more climbing per day than LEJOG. It was going to be epic. We were doing this for charity to remember our neighbour and friend Jonathan Curwen, who passed away last year due to stomach cancer, at the age of 42. Find out more details in the epilogue.

A Long and Winding Road
The lessons from my big cycling adventure
(giving up was never an option)

There were many lessons that I took away from the experience that can be applied to most situations in life and business.

1. Defining an end destination will spur you on to do better

Having a clear destination and direction of travel really helped to focus the mind. I found that having an end point to get to each day help me focus and I actually got more energy as I approached the end. Without a clearly defined end point you can easily meander, drift or be overwhelmed by the whole event. The same principle applies to providing a clear vision for teams. Build the end vision with your team and keep checking that you're still on track.

2. Break the day / tasks down into digestible chunks

You can easily be overwhelmed by the size of the task / the day ahead. So, break your day down into mini goals. I would stop 2-3 times a day so that I was cycling for around 2 hours at a time. This also helped to refuel the body and mind. I always recommend breaking down large projects /

programmes into smaller deliverables - eat the elephant one bite at a time.

3. Don't burn yourself out / Go at your own pace / pace yourself

Don't be tempted to burn yourself out, as it catches up with you, and you end up not working to your full potential. This happened on day 6 when I climbed the Kirkstone Pass in the Lake District and did a fair bit of climbing in the morning. I went too hard and overdid it and it caught up with me later in the day. I struggled in the last 3rd of the day from Gretna Green to Moffat. Establish your pace and if you are doing endurance events stick to the pace you are comfortable with.

4. Be reasonably scientific about how you will achieve your goal but experiment to get better results

I estimated the calories that I would need to take on, given the calories I was using. I based this on my training rides. However, I realised that even though I had upped my mileage that I was not losing any weight. During the big ride I learned what was right for me and ended up eating more normal food, rather than energy bars and energy gels. I also stopped using caffeine gels as they were pushing my heart rate artificially high and instead would have a can of full fat coke a day instead.

So there is a lot to be said for planning but in the end experimentation does get better results (and helped lose some weight, as it is easier to carry less weight around).

5. Really steep hills (and difficult tasks) require certain coping techniques

I climbed over 44,000 feet over the 10 days and climbed some pretty big hills. However, it wasn't until day 9 that I realised how to properly deal with them. I therefore focused on a spot 8-10 feet in front of me, stayed seated, did not hunch up and maintained a cycling rhythm (a cadence that was comfortable and got me up the hill without too much effort). This worked a treat, as I did not focus on the hill. Before I knew it, I was at the top of the hill and accelerating and moving up the gears up more gradual inclines. I still use this technique today and it works every time, as standing up to climb hills gets you out of puff pretty quickly and catches you out later.

You can employ a similar approach to difficult tasks – break the task down and grind out the answer by focusing on what is in front of you, rather than being overwhelmed by the larger challenge ahead of you.

6. Listen to your body and feed it

It sounds pretty obvious but water and food are required to fuel you and keep you alert. On day 3 (leaving Bristol), when it was raining, I was pretty miserable and I forgot to drink enough. I ended up dehydrated and was completely washed out after the first 30 of the 85 miles to be completed on the day. But after refuelling and topping up on water I was revitalised.

On the penultimate day (just outside of Tain), when I was just 5 miles from the end of the day (although it was a 119-mile day) I hit the wall with chronic neck pain and a lack of energy. I stopped, rested, stretched and put fuel in my body to finish the day.

This lessons applies to everyday life – listen to your body and feed it and make sure you are hydrated.

7. Step away from the problem, regroup and then tackle it

On some of the big hills (especially just outside of Drumnadrochit) they almost seemed impossible to climb. Occasionally I would stop at the bottom or mid-way through to let my heart rate fall back to a resting rate and to regather myself. However, I did cycle every mile of the 975.

There is no shame in stopping / taking a break to achieve your goals. You can still achieve the end goal without killing yourself. Really steep hills (and difficult tasks) require certain coping techniques. You don't always need to rush to achieve your goals.

8. Your mental resolve defines you especially in the face of obstacles

Cycling 100 miles a day, day after day meant that my body and mind were tired. The weather was also very testing at times. When faced with these challenges you can take a few choices:

1. Just keep going, deal with it and grind out the hard yards

2. Take a break to reframe the problem or re-energise yourself

3. Give up (this was never an option on the ride)

The same options present themselves when running projects and programmes. Unforeseen problems crop up regularly and deadlines need to be met. Perseverance and taking a step back to reframe the problem can help to ensure you deliver the outcomes for the programme.

9. Use all the tools and support available to do your best

I used the following tools and support to ensure I did my best:

- I used energy gels, energy bars, Ibuprofen and regularly massaged my legs to get the best performance over the journey.

- My father was my support vehicle and would make me meals and look after my bike, so that I could focus solely on cycling.

- I used a Garmin Edge Explorer 820 as my navigation tool.

- I used a Garmin Vivoactive HR watch to monitor my distance, speed and heart rate.

- The support of family and friends gave me words of encouragement that really helped during the tough times.

Don't be scared of using all the tools at your disposal to deliver the best results.

10. Local knowledge beats any in depth (outsider) research

On 3 days I ignored my well laid plans and went with the superior knowledge of a local. Those 3 days were better for listening to and heeding the local knowledge. For example – I had a tour of South Shropshire and Shrewsbury on Day 4. On day 6 I did some serious but stunning hill climbing in the Lake District, rather than spending a lot of the day on an A road. On Day 7 I avoided a monster hill outside of Moffat, in Scotland, and instead took in a much more scenic route that was longer but more manageable.

When delivering projects or programmes get the local insights / engage local stakeholders in order to deliver better outcomes.

11. Give yourself some downtime

Although I was focused on getting to an end point, this singular focus also allowed me the time and space to think about many other things in my life. In some ways it was a near religious experience as it brought everything else into focus.

Have you ever wondered why some of your best ideas happen in the shower? This will be one of the few opportunities where you allow your brain some down time.

In our lives, we are often too busy to give ourselves the space to think. Try to ensure that you are not a "busy fool" as downtime regularly pays back with moments of inspiration.

12. Life is about the journey and not just the end destination. Enjoy the ride!

I could have completely focused on the end destination and on occasions when I was tired or soaking wet that was required, but I fully embraced the journey.

I took lots of photos, kept a diary, used the time to reflect and enjoyed the scenery and the experience. Too often the end point is seen as the be all and end all. It doesn't need to be like that. Enjoy the journey on the way to your goal.

The big cycling adventure has been a life changing experience for me. It was amazing.

Epilogue: The Jonathan Curwen Memorial ride around Wales

I met my neighbour Jonathan Curwen when they moved into the new housing development we live on, back in 2012. Jonathan, Vicky and his lovely 3 children lived across the road from us. We got to know each other well and our children grew up playing together.

Jonathan moved away to a new house in September 2017. Unfortunately, at the same time Jonathan was diagnosed with stomach cancer. He went through all of the treatments and surgery later that year and early the following year. I went to see Jonathan in hospital in Liverpool. The surgery that he had was a major operation, but he was in good spirits. That was the last time that I saw Jonathan.

Although he was given the all clear a few months later the cancer returned and he passed away almost 12 months to the day of the initial diagnosis. It was a real shock and it was terrible that his life had been taken away at the age of 42, leaving Vicky and 3 children under 10 behind.

It affected me (Jonathan was 4 years younger than me) and my other friends. Over the Christmas period we decided that we should do something big to remember him and to raise funds for the Clatterbridge Cancer trust. Clatterbridge looked after Jonathan during his illness. We decided that we would cycle around Wales. It sounds easy when you say it quickly!

The planning began on New Years' Day. I planned the route and even provisionally booked rooms. 4 of us were going to take on the challenge: me, Jez Scaiff, Paul Evans and Ben Willis. Jez lives in Tarporley, is a keen cyclist and is the friend that joined me for a day on the LEJOG trip. Paul is a friend I had met several years ago on holiday. He is a good cyclist and joined me for half a day on LEJOG. Ben is mine and Jonathan's old neighbour and a good friend. Ben has next to no cycling experience, but is generally as fit as a butchers' dog.

My dad, William Lyon, agreed to be our support vehicle again. He was keen to get involved and help out.

This was another big ride. Almost 100 miles per day, but much hillier than LEJOG. It was going to be interesting cycling with 3 friends as I was quite accustomed to cycling on my own. The training was more intensive than LEJOG as I had learned that I needed to get the miles in the legs much earlier.

The week's riding was awesome. The team spirit and friendship was just brilliant. We helped each other immensely and learned how to ride together and work as a team. Here are the highlights of the ride:

- Ben lost his phone on the first leg of the first day. Thankfully his son Dylan was able to locate it via the find my phone app.

- We got horribly lost in Cardiff and didn't get to the hotel until 8.45pm
- The Wye valley was amazingly beautiful, we followed the river for miles and had a break at Tintern abbey
- 3 punctures (2 for Jez and one for Paul). I managed not to get any on either LEJOG or the Wales ride.
- Seeing Nick and Kerry Farren on the Gower peninsula. Clatterbridge helped to save Kerry's life.
- Jez's incredible navigation skills, without a sat nav and a map, he still found us the biggest hills but got us where we needed to be.
- Ben's incredible fitness. He is not a cyclist but got stronger and stronger as the week went on.
- Paul's very funny catchphrases / comments. One of his funniest, as we were approaching Tenby, as I was cursing Jez for taking us up ridiculous hills was "just kick him in the slats". I almost fell off my bike laughing.
- The stunning countryside / coastline of Wales – it was a pleasure to be cycling in such wonderful scenery.
- The intense heat (yes, in Wales!) and the headwinds that meant we were putting in 50% more effort than we would be doing normally.
- Jez's knee wasn't in good shape on one day which meant that he was on my back wheel for most of that day.
- The incredible generosity of people along the way and via the power of Facebook. It helped to keep our spirits high.

- The support that we received from our families, both before the ride (as the training is quite a commitment) and during the ride. It meant so much to have our families behind us.
- Racing on Anglesey – we had already covered 550 miles, but found energy from somewhere to race up the (many) hills of Anglesey.
- Mark Cotton and Mark Hammond's support, to bring us in on the final leg of the ride.
- My dad's amazing food and drink, company, pool skills and the unforgettable nest of tables.
- The welcoming committee at the Tirley Garth Garden Fete. We were all overwhelmed and a little bit emotional.

Here are the vital statistics from the Jonathan Curwen Memorial ride around Wales.

Day	Start	End	Elevation	Mins	Miles	Cumulative
1	Tarporley	Llandrindod Wells	4,046	383	102	102
2	Llandrindod Wells	Cardiff	5,729	460	112	215
3	Cardiff	Tenby	6,156	469	104	318
4	Tenby	Aberaeron	7,131	476	100	419
5	Aberaeron	Abergynolwyn	4,533	316	66	485
6	Abergynolwyn	Amlwch	5,124	405	86	571
7	Amlwch	Tarporley	3,642	412	96	667
Total			36,361	2,921	667	
Average per day			5,194	417	95	

The most important thing about the ride was that we were able to raise just over £4,500 for the Clatterbridge Cancer charity. I am sure that Jonathan would have been proud of the immense effort that his friends put in to raise money for such a good cause.

Maps of the epic ride

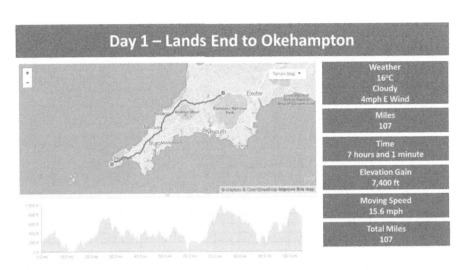

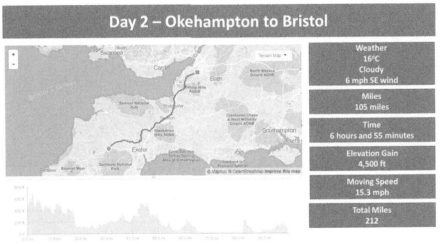

Day 3 – Bristol to Leominster

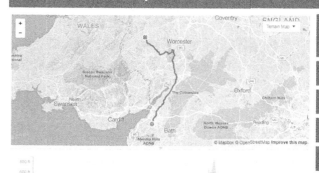

Weather 14°C Heavy Rain 8 mph E wind	
Miles 85	
Time 6 hours and 11 minutes	
Elevation Gain 3,386 ft	
Moving Speed 14.2 mph	
Total Miles 297	

Day 4 – Leominster to Tarporley

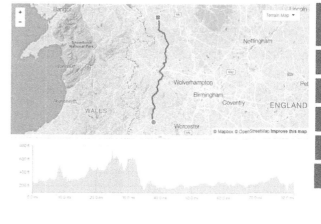

Weather 12°C, Heavy Rain, 4 mph NW wind	
Miles 80 miles	
Time 5 hours and 24 minutes	
Elevation Gain 3,087 ft	
Moving Speed 15.1 mph	
Total Miles 377	

Day 5 – Tarporley to Bowness

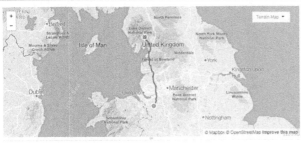

Weather
16°C
Cloudy
12 mph NW wind

Miles
100

Time
6 hours and 25 minutes

Elevation Gain
3,852 ft

Moving Speed
15.8 mph

Total Miles
477

Day 6 – Bowness to Moffat

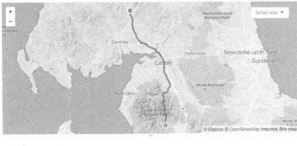

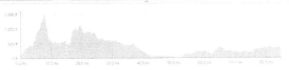

Weather
16°C
Cloudy
16 mph W wind

Miles
89

Time
6 hours

Elevation Gain
4,852 ft

Moving Speed
15.1 mph

Total Miles
566

Day 7 – Moffat to Perth

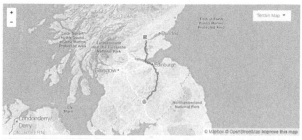

Weather 10°C Very Wet 7 mph E wind	
Miles 107	
Time 7 hours and 49 minutes	
Elevation Gain 4,790 ft	
Moving Speed 14.0 mph	
Total Miles 673	

Day 8 – Perth to Kinlochleven

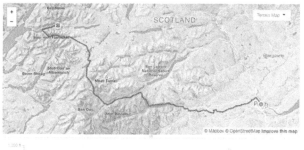

Weather 14°C Sunny 7 mph E wind	
Miles 95	
Time 6 hours and 15 minutes	
Elevation Gain 3,832 ft	
Moving Speed 15.7 mph	
Total Miles 768	

Day 9 – Kinlochleven to Tain

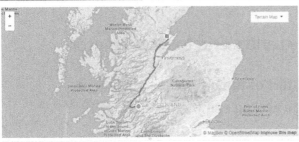

Weather
21°C
Wet and Sunny
15 mph W wind

Miles
119

Time
7 hours and 48 minutes

Elevation Gain
3,898 ft

Moving Speed
15.4 mph

Total Miles
887

Day 10 – Tain to John O'Groats

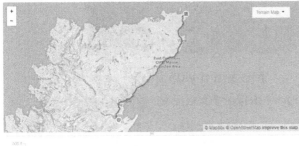

Weather
14°C
Sunny
7 mph E wind

Miles
88

Time
6 hours and 4 minutes

Elevation Gain
4,806 ft

Moving Speed
14.8 mph

Total Miles
975

Photos of the Epic Ride

Day 1 – Land's End to Okehampton

At the start of the big cycling adventure.
Let the cycling commence!! Boom!!!

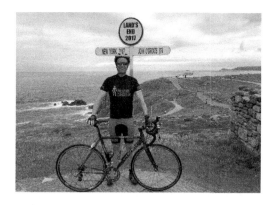

Me and my dad,
my trusty support driver for the long journey ahead.

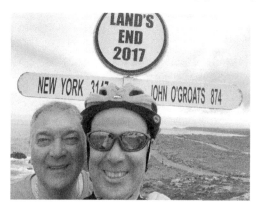

St Michaels Mount, after about 15 miles.

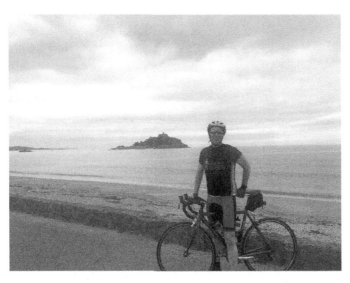

A café North of Wadebridge with an inspiring name!

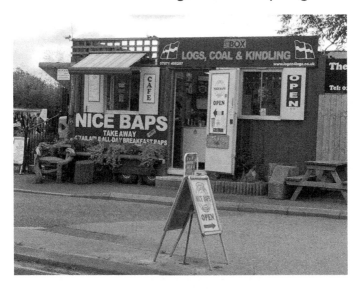

Launceston Castle.

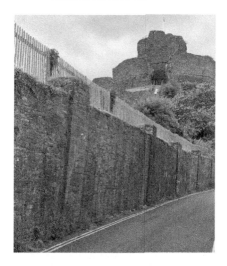

The main square in Launceston.
They'd even got the bunting out for me!

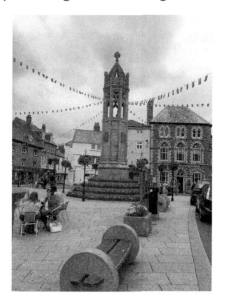

Leaving Cornwall at last.

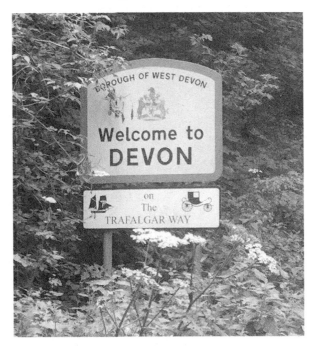

Bum Cream dispenser, courtesy of my good friends Martin and Sue at the end of Day 1.

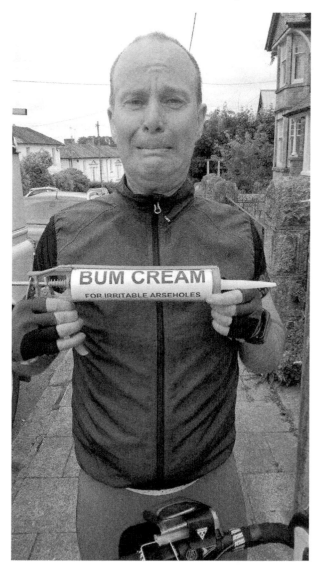

Day 2 – Okehampton to Bristol

The friendly cows of Devon coming out to offer their support.

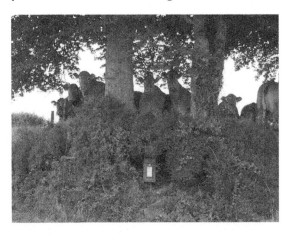

Stretching out (in a layby, not the road).

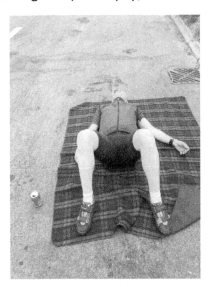

Bristol marina from outside The Cottage Inn.

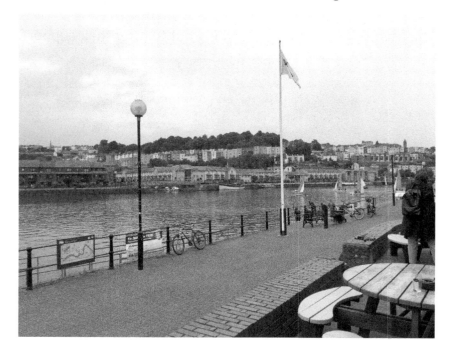

Brilliant street art in Bristol on the way back from dinner.

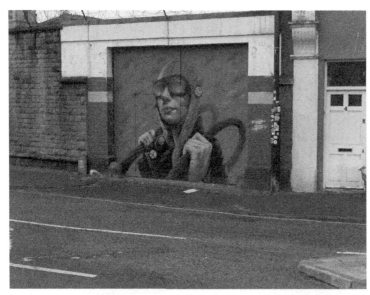

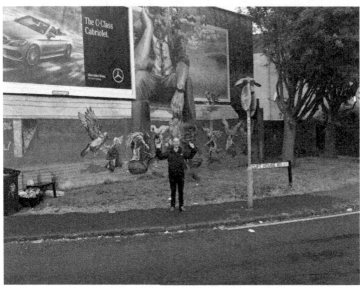

Day 3 – Bristol to Leominster

Ashton Gate Stadium (Bristol City Football Club).

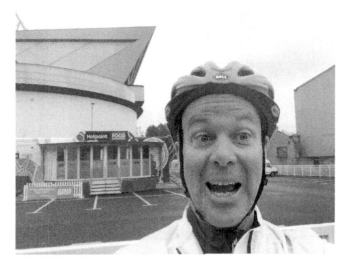

Clifton Suspension Bridge. Very wet.

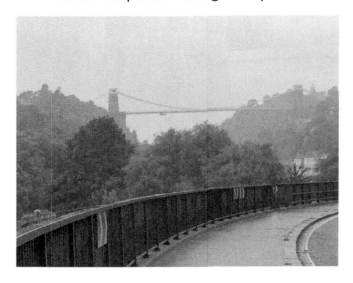

Bristol Cathedral. Lovely, but still wet.

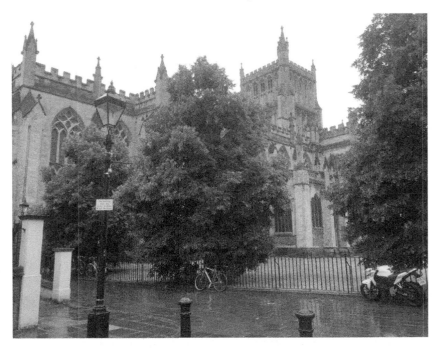

A steep hill in Bristol. I'm not going up that.

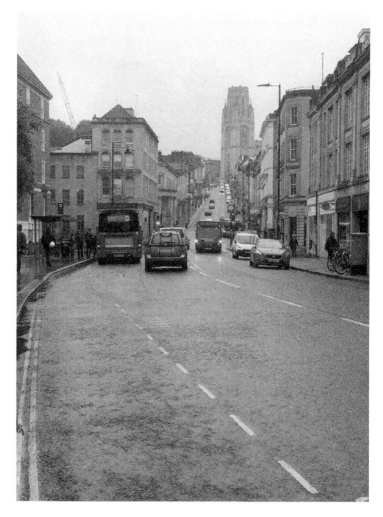

The Malvern Hills.

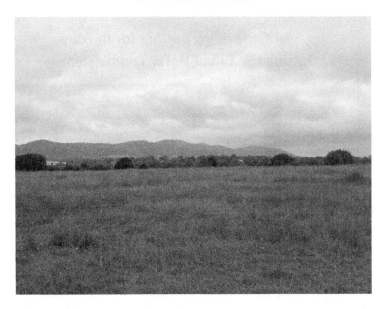

Day 4 – Leominster to Tarporley

Jez Scaiff, my riding partner for the day.
Outside the Talbot Hotel, Leominster.

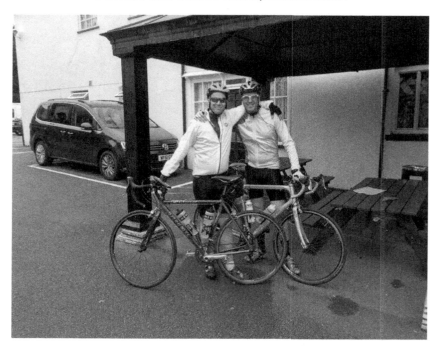

The Welcoming Committee on Tarporley High Street.

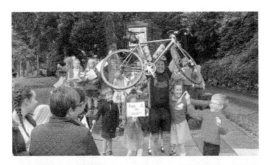

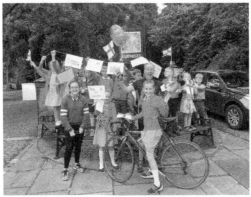

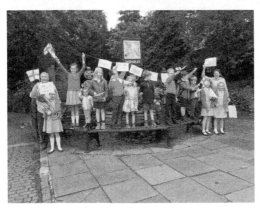

Day 5 – Tarporley to Bowness

Ready to go on Day 5 with Helen seeing me off from home.

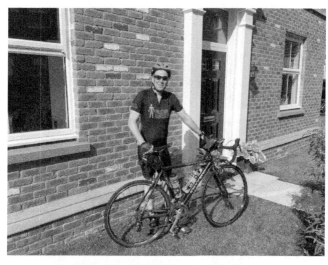

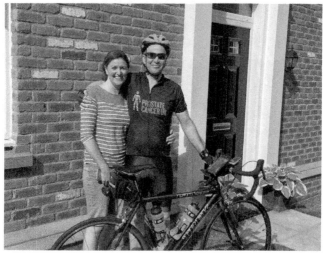

The Halliwell Jones stadium.
Home to Warrington Wolves rugby league club.

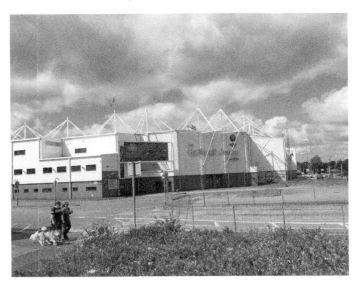

The Bucks Head, Abram, Wigan.
Loved the sign that appears to offer free beer?!?

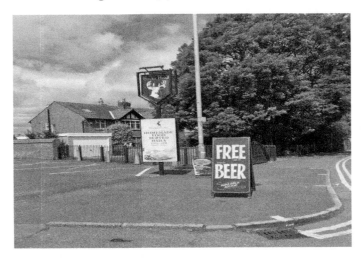

Lancaster, Greaves Park.
Check out Dad's home-made brew box.

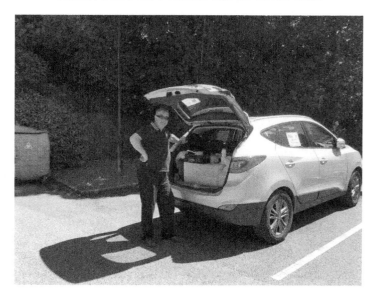

Lovely scenery at Milnthorpe.

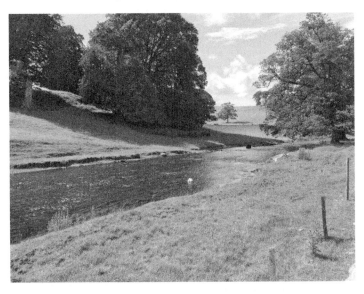

A heron at Milnthorpe.

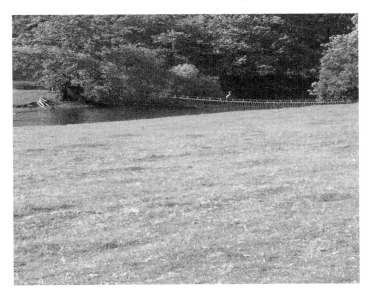

Early views of the Lake District.

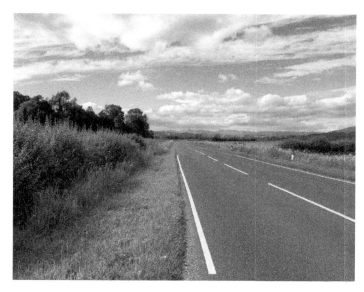

A lovely evening in Windermere.

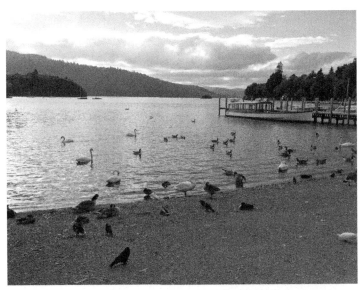

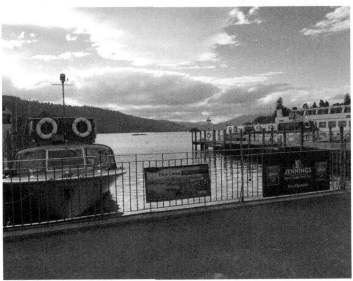

Day 6 – Bowness to Moffat

Ready to go on Day 6
with Paul "King of the Mountains" Evans.

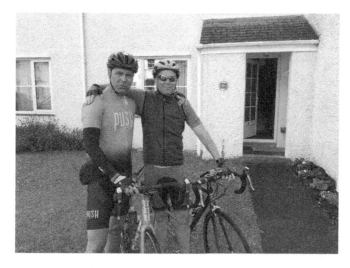

A lovely spot by Ullswater, before the climbing.

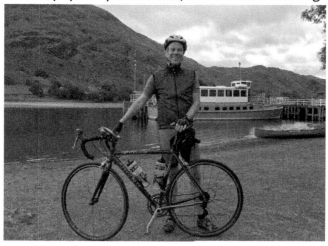

Views from the Kirkstone Pass.

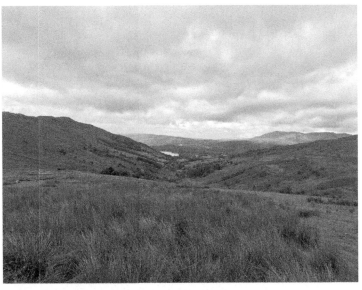

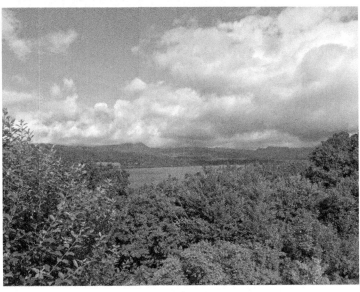

At the top of the Kirkstone pass – we made it!

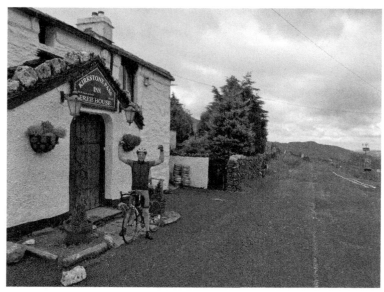

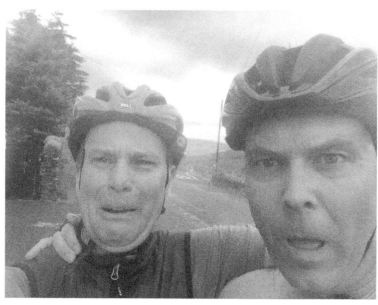

Paul Evans leaving me in Carlisle.

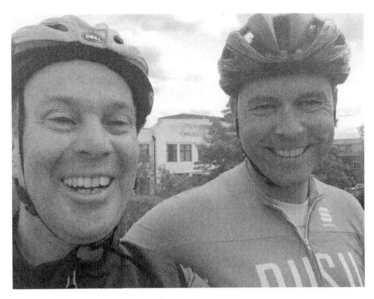

Carlisle Castle.

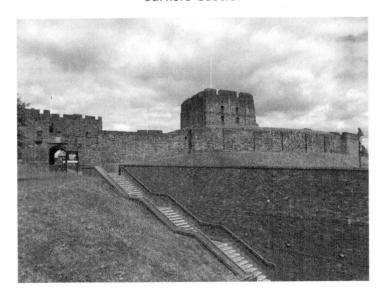

Scotland!

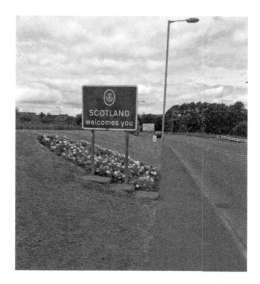

Gretna Green. Still a long way to go!

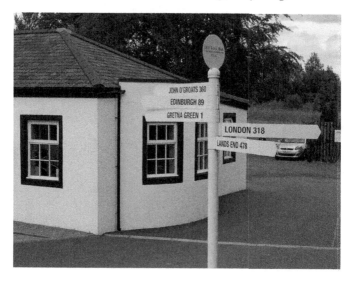

The famous earless ram of Moffat.

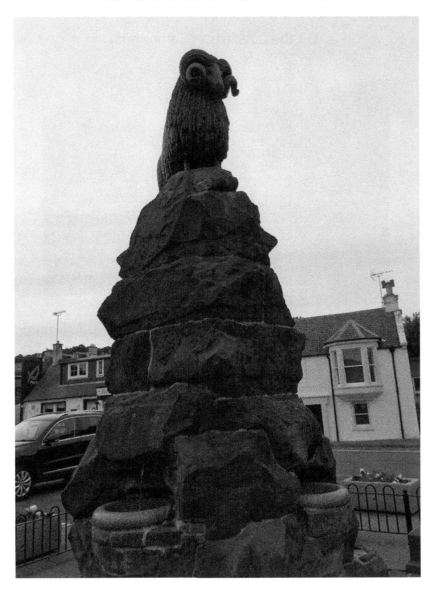

Day 7 – Moffat to Perth

On the outskirts of Edinburgh.

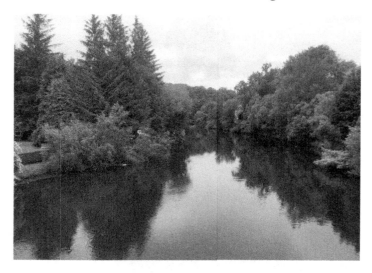

Views of the Forth Bridges.

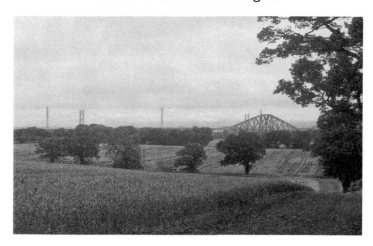

Forth new and old road bridges – very windy and unsettling.

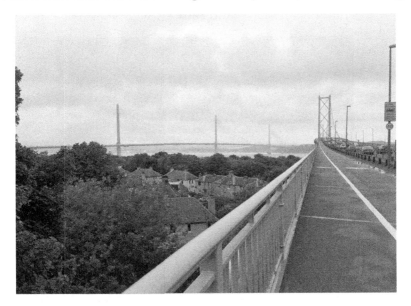

The Forth Bridge.

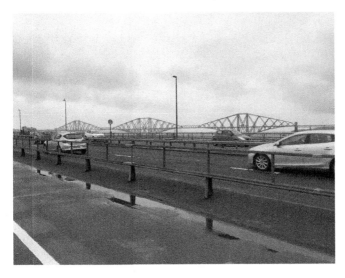

Evidence that my face got completely battered by the wind and rain.

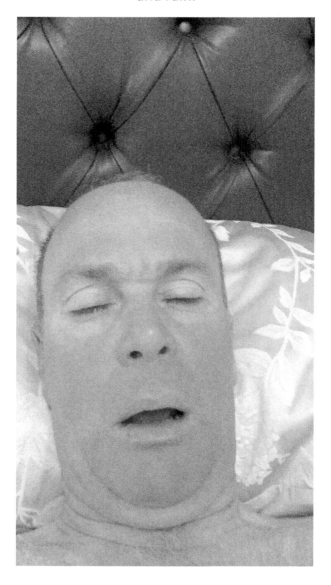

Day 8 – Perth to Kinlochleven

Dad looking cool by Loch Earn, but those shorts look a bit tight.

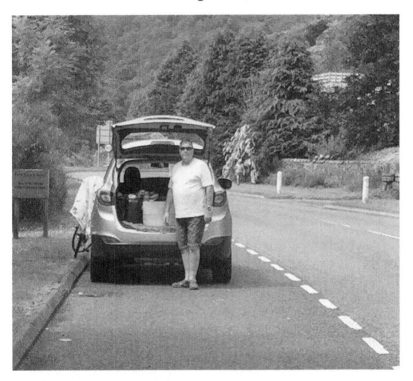

Lovely scenery at Loch Earn.

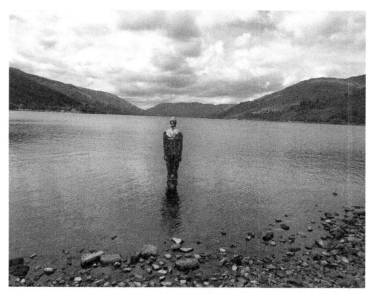

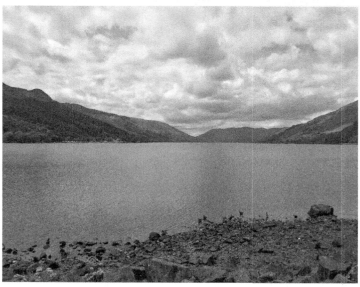

Lovely scenery all around.

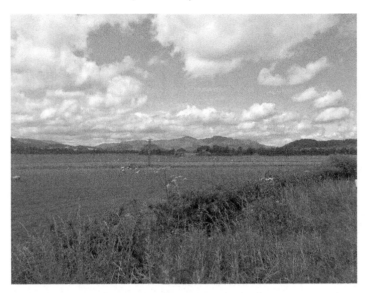

First distillery (and oldest) spotted so far.

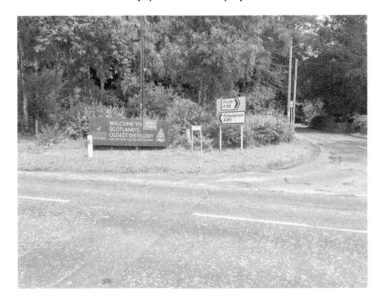

The view from Crieff – it's going to get lumpy.

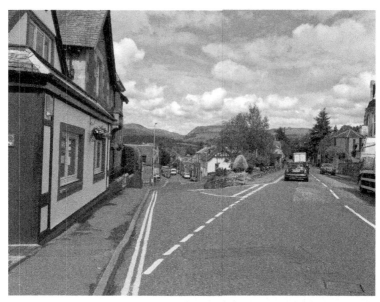

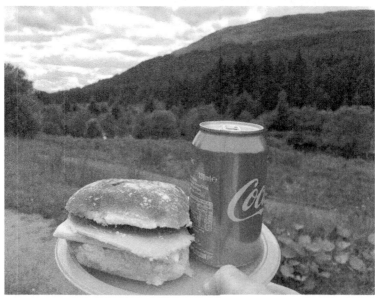

Stunning scenery on the A85.

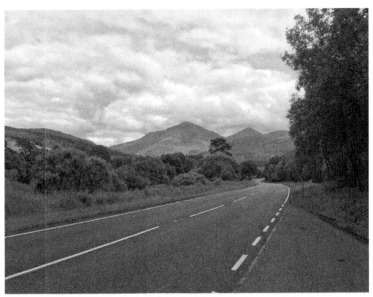

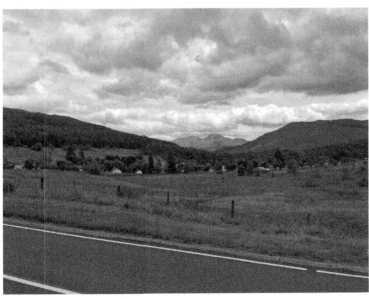

More stunning scenery on the A85.

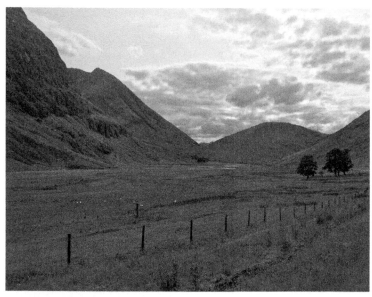

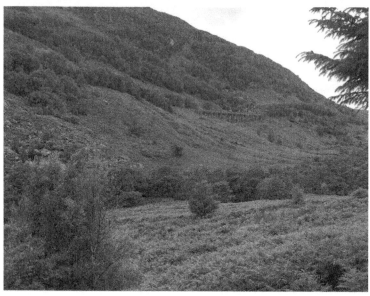

More stunning scenery on the A85.

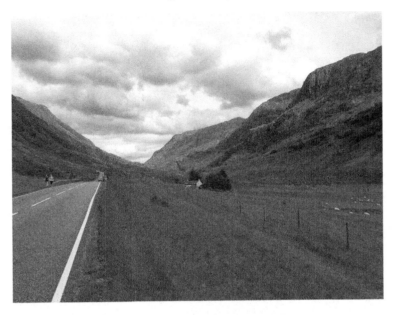

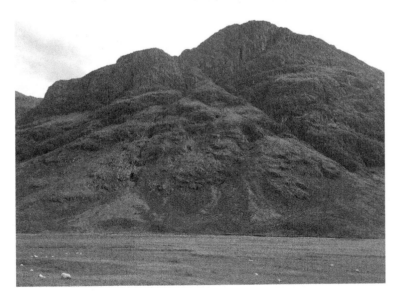

Entering the Highlands.

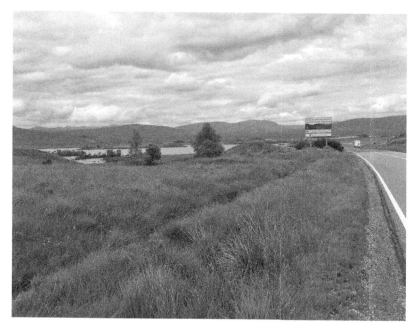

A lovely evening at the Onich Hotel, overlooking Loch Linnhe.

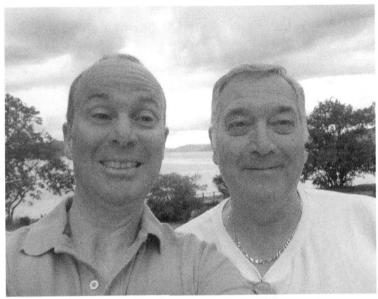

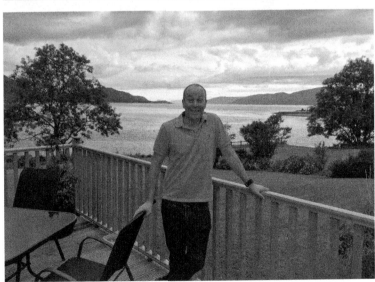

Day 9 – Kinlochleven to Tain

Invergarry Bridge. Not raining!

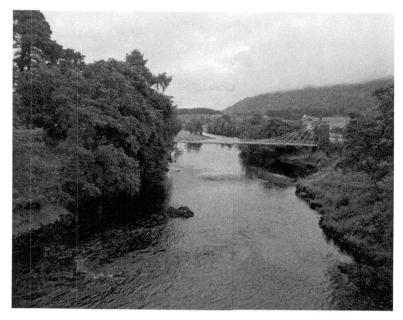

Urquhart castle on the banks of Loch Ness.

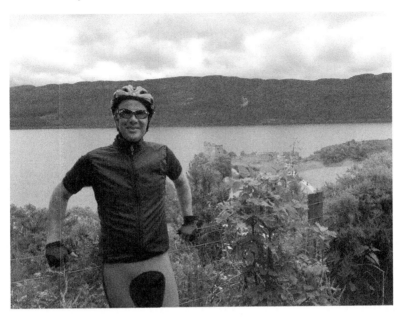

Day 10 – Tain to John O'Groats

Not far now!

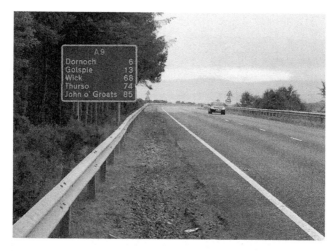

Fellow LEJOG riders, who also saw Tom Jones, the night before us, in Cartmel!

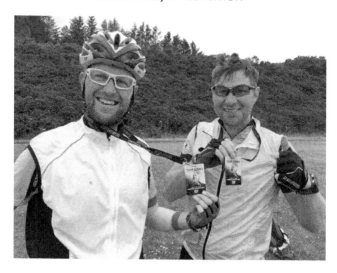

The lovely little village of Brora.

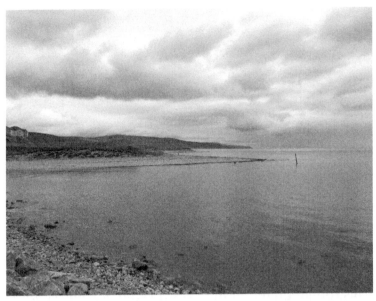

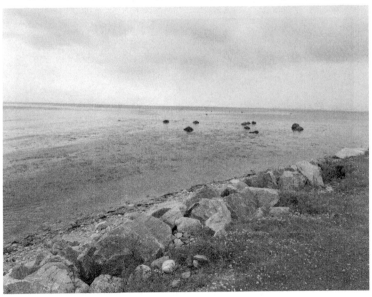

Looking back to Dunrobin Castle.

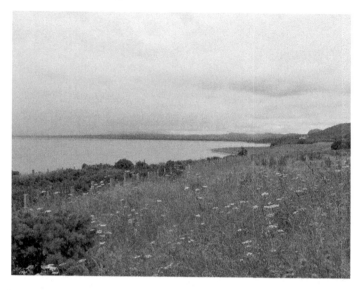

This reminded me of my ex-colleague, Rachel Mound!

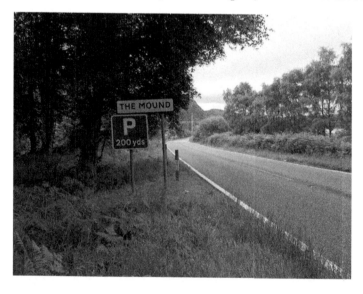

The End - A proud, proud moment!

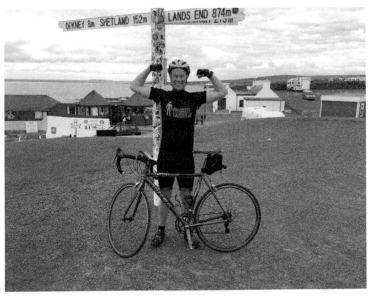

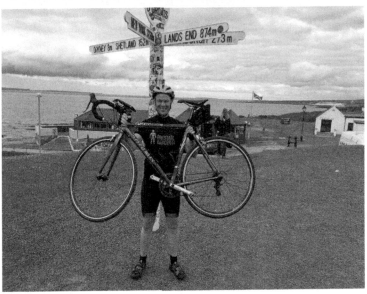

A proud moment for the Lyon family.

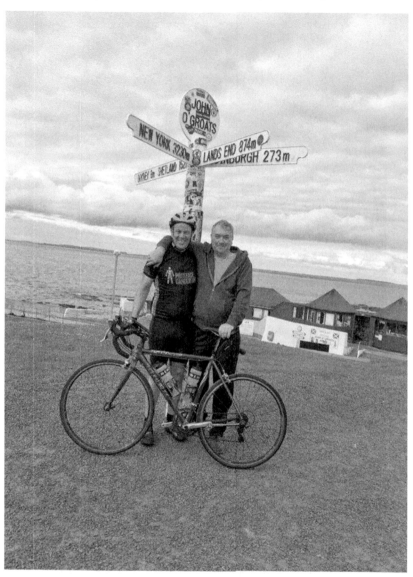

Printed in Great Britain
by Amazon